I0412781

Living Life As
A Cancer Survivor

Living Life As
A Cancer Survivor

Rebecca A. Kuffour

Copyright © 2011 by Rebecca A. Kuffour.

ISBN: Softcover   978-1-4653-7739-5

All rights reserved. No part of this book may be reproduced or transmitted in any form or by any means, electronic or mechanical, including photocopying, recording, or by any information storage and retrieval system, without permission in writing from the copyright owner.

This book was printed in the United States of America.

To order additional copies of this book, contact:
Xlibris Corporation
1-888-795-4274
www.Xlibris.com
Orders@Xlibris.com
105925

CHAPTER 1

Imagine that you have been told that you have breast cancer for the first time in your life and you just gave birth to your third child not too long a go "thinking it's your last one", you might be;

(A) Crying your heart out and wondering "Why me out of all the people in the world!"

(B) Going delusional thinking that your children are going to be mother-less and life-less without you.

(C) Completely fainting or staring straight through the wall seeing your life flashing before your eyes.

-OR-

(D) All of the above.

But to understand the feeling and the journey it took for me to realize how life would change from bold to abnormal you'll have to know it all started in the year 2000 in Ohio where my husband at the time and I lived with our two children and I was pregnant with our third child. After having our child I started to feel pain in my right arm. During the time my newly born daughter was only four months old when it started. It was painful to the point that we had to see a doctor, to know what was going on with me. Come to find out it was breast cancer in my right breast and in the lymph nod. After the discovery of my cancer, the doctor tried to give us some advice on seeing a therapist to understand more about the cancer and how it will affect my life, and family. When talking to my therapist, he explained the steps of chemotherapy, medication I would have to take including the ups and Downs of the whole situation. The next two weeks we went to see a surgeon to talk about the next steps of this ***undesired piece of a puzzle*** and what he would be able to do to try to get rid of it. He even explained what I should expect after the surgery during the removal of my breast and how I would feel. Also explained that I would be going through a cycle of pain in my breast and arm, the pain was more than I'd expect it to be. It was so unbearable to the point that I could not do anything, like for example; going to the bathroom by my self and even bathing myself properly. My mother, sister and also my friends were the ones who help me and "sometime my husband." But it wasn't til I came home that I notice how hard it was going to be on me and my family mental and physically especially when it came to my children. As I struggled to walk through the doors of our home with my mother and friend by my side as phsyical support, I caught my oldest daughter staring at me as if I was a stranger born as a mutant. I wasn't so shocked knowing that this wasn't their usually greeting. Their regular greets always started with them racing towards me and give huges and kisses, but it seemed liked they didn't want anything to do with me, as if I was spreading a contagious virus, like I was worth-less. It was kind of hard not to show sadness in front of them due to the shameful pain that ran through out my body without going to the emergency room once a week.

I was heart broken and stress out hoping another momment wouldn't change me or cause this experience to go even more wrong. But I guess I was wrong . . . . especially when it came time to doing chemothearpy, my hair started to fall out of place so I had to shave my head fully bald, So my husband did. As I felt the blade slide up and down my sclap *I felt tears crawling from my eyes, it was like I lost the few thing that made me a Women,* it's one of the moments I'll never forget.

As I was still going through this painful experience with my family, my church "Assemblies of God" even offered to lend a helping hand to me with prayers and money. Sometimes I would go to church on weekdays to say a few prayers or I would pray at home. In church I would feel so sick around people that I'd have to go home and in other cases it was that I felt bad about me not having any hair on my head which would cause me to look around at people's hair dos and say to myself "Wish it was possible for me to be normal again."

After five years of *struggling with this heavy black burden hanging over my shoulders,* I discover that I was cancer free (thank God). When I found out that I was cancer free, I decided to go to church to give my testimony. It was a way of letting people know what I've been going through and how the lord has cured me from cancer. And also how wonderful and power the lord can be and if you follow him he will create miracles full of joy and happiness.

CHAPTER 2

After I was cancer free I started working at home doing hair, which lasted only for a few months. So I decide to look for a new job, that was when my husband and I started to have problems. I started to pray and ask god to please help me find a job and move out. My prays was answered, I finally found a job to help my husband pay the bills and did what a wife was suppose to do at home, I cleaned the house, watched the kids, fed them and also cook. Then one day I said to myself; that something wasn't right about my husband because he would sometimes come home from work with another pair of clothing on. It made me wonder if there was another women in the picture. Then one Sunday after church, we came home and the phone rung, my husband answer the phone and it was another women on the phone, so I went upstairs to pick up the other line to hear what they were talking about. They were talking about him buying a car. I was so up set that I cursed at both of them and I hanged up the phone. As soon as I went down stairs I asked him who was that other women he was talking to, he wouldn't tell me who she was, so it resulted in us having a big argument and our relationship was over. That's when I decided to move back to New York city.

When I moved back to New York, I was so lucky that my boss at the time had talked to my supervisor about me coming back to New York to work.

So my supervisor gave me a second chance to come back and work at Long Island College Hospital. When it came to finding a place to live in New York, my children and I were living with my oldest sister Joyce in Brooklyn for about 7 months. Later, My children and I decided to move and get our own apartment. After a few years passed by *full of loneliness,* I met a wonderful guy that I knew before I met my husband and we became friends. Later on when we learned more about each other we both decided to date. During that time I couldn't have any more children. Luckily, god created another miracle. I had a beautiful baby boy, who I called my miracle baby. After giving birth to my son, I knew our family was finally complete. Then I decided to tie my tubes. Now our family was completed.

CHAPTER 3

Then one day, I went to the doctors office to do blood work, which I did every 6 months a check up, but that day *there was a black cloud over my head*, the next week my doctor called me to let me know that the blood work came back positive and that the lab found cancer in my blood, so she wanted me to do another blood work to see if the second one will come back the same, it did so my doctor told me that I will have to do some test from my back and other test and I did it the answer came, it was breast cancer.

That day I was in my car when the doctor called me to give me the news. I had to stop the car and put it on park because I was terrify so I started to cry my kids asked me what is wrong with me, I couldn't tell them what was going on with me at that moment, things was just running through my head right away, I told my self that my god is in control.

After all that we both sat down to discuss about me doing chemotherapy with her but I decided not to do so. Mainly because my cousin and I had a discussion about doing my treatment at New York Presbyterian hospital. So I should talk to my doctor about transfer my record to the new doctor office. Before that I got sick and was drove to the hospital by my cousin, who works with me. Through that I was recommend to a wonderful doctor who is specialize in breast cancer. We had an appointment to see the doctor to discussed about my history and treatment. that was when my new doctor told me and my cousin that it was breast cancer gone to the liver. That day it was a nightmare for us. I didn't know what to say or do. All I did was cry my heart out and ask my self why me. Why do this have to happen to me and my family. I cry all the way home that day. When I came home I didn't know how to tell my children and family, but somewhere in my heart I know that god will help me through it. It was so hard for me at work so I couldn't ever think right. ALL I would do is just cry and pray and say god please let me live to see my children 's growth and wise success through out the future.

CHAPTER 4

A week later my cousin and I want back to see the doctor to talked about treatment and what stage the cancer was in. When he told us that the cancer was at stage four. I started to cry more and say how can this cancer be at stage four. Then the doctor ask me how many children do I have and if I was married. It because he wanted to tell me that I would need to do a surgery, which was

going to be a hysterectomy. through that I won't be able to conceive again. It was okay with me because of my condition

The day of my surgery it was so sad for me because I felt like I was alone and wasn't coming back. I felt like I was going to leave my children behind But the lord did not let it happen. My brother came home from Iraq the week that I was going to have my surgery done. So my mother said to him drive Rebecca to the hospital about four o'clock in the morning. But my surgery was for five o'clock. I was so scaret while I was by my self. So I said a little pray asking god to free me and let me come back save.

During the time of my surgery my mother couldn't be there for me because she had to be home with my children. So when after the surgery was done it took so long for me to come back to my self. When I finally came to my self the only family that was there was my cousin and her husband. They were the only people that I see which made me so happy because I knew that somebody care for me.

I was in so much pain that I could even talk, walk or even get up from bed. I had to ask a nurse to please wash me up. I could eat until the next day. The surgeons came to see how I was doing after the surgery and asked me if I was in pain. I answer yes I 'am in pain. They ask me if I would like to go home and I said yes. The next day they came to see me again and said to me you are going home. I was so happy to go home to my beautiful children. The doctor give me an appointment to come back to see him just to see if everything was right with me.

After I came home from the hospital. I called my doctor so that I can be schedule for an appointment for the next three weeks. So he gave me a day to come and I went for my checkup. the following month I call my chemotherapy doctor so that I can star my treatment as soon as possible he told me that I will have to be heal first. So when I was heal I went back to do my treatment for the first time.

CHAPTER 5

The chemotherapy that I was about to do name is trastuzumab the other name for this medication is herceptin. This type of medication is to treat certain types of breast cancer. herceptin is use to attaches the cancer cells and also in other immune cell to help kill them. The herceptin is given to me by infusion me in the vein. The first dose was given to me for about ninety minutes and from that day I have bring receiving it for thirty minutes, The dose depend on your weight.

The first side effect that I got from this medicine is feeling ligtheaded and dizzy headache, shortness of breath. It came a time at work that I felt so dizzy and lightheaded that I end up fainting in the kitchen at my work place so I ended up in the emergency room. It was because of my blood pressure was so high that they couldn't take me up to a room. until my pressure came down. I had to stay for two days in the hospital. Come to find out my heart play a part in it.

So because of all these problems my doctor always lets me do test for my heart, chest, and also do CTS, MRI, and also blood work and stress test every three month. It came to a time that I had to stop the treatment for sometime. Then later I went back to it again. With this treatment I'am tired sometime weak. I even lost my appetite.

CHAPTER 6

Now the medicine I'am taking is also helping me but I get a bad side effect from it The name of the medicine is arimidex. The other name is anastrozole. Taking medicine is very helpful to me. But the side effect is painful for me. I'am always having aches and pain. Sometime I `can even climb the step because I be so tired and also can sleep. So my doctor prescribe a medicatine for me to sleep

But sometime I will think that by me taking this medicatine to sleep I will not be able to wake up again. That was one of my biggest fear. One day my doctor recommend that I see a therapist to help me cope with the cancer and to talk to them about what I'am going through.

The threapist that is working with me is a male therapist he is so nice and friendly. He is always willing to listen to what I have to say. We discuss about so many things like my life my childern and also the cancer and the support that I;am get from my family and friend and also my son father. Which I call my husband.

My therapist helps me to overcome my biggest fear and it was going to sleep and not waking up again. It was scary that I can think that way, When I think about me going to sleep not waking up is very sad. So all I can do is just cry my heart out and ask god to watch over me. Sometime at night I will sit on my bed and call the name of the lord and say. Why this sickness did chose me.

Any time my therapist ask me about the cancer I cry. I know that one day this sickness will take me on a journey. Some where I never been before that where I will never see my four beautiful kids again. It sad to say that knowing that your life will one day end. Sometime I ask my self will I grow old or will this sickness kill me.

The one thing that I always talk about with my therapist is how strong my belief is with god and when you lean on him he will create so many miracles in your life. I also tell him that god was the one who help me through all this by me praying and fasting.

CHAPTER 7

ONE day in the hospital I had a beautiful dream that I saw god with my mother and the devil. God and my mother was dressed in white from head to toe. The devil was dressed in black. All three of them were standing in line by my hospital room door. God was first, my mother was second, and the devil was third. God said to my mother " you can go in to see your child but the devil will not come in. That day I knew I can over come every obstacle that comes my way.

IT is easy for anybody to say what they want to say until they put there feet into your shoes. That's when they will know what pain you are facing and feeling. Only those who wearn my shoes know what I'm going through.

As a person going through cancer it is very hard sometime I can even think straight. With all these things going through my mind it seens like just yesterday my doctor told me that I'm diagnose with cancer. When I think about the frist day I cry.

I say how can this happen to a good person like me for me to say that then you know I'm facing. I will be laydown and start to talk to my self like if I 'm crazy. this will make you go out of your mind.

CHAPTER 8

From time to time I think if I was to die what will my childern do or say about their mother. I sometime say to my self will they miss me or will they remember all the good time we spened together and the wonderful things we did together.

I always think about me dieing and when I'm gone what will happen to them. Will they be treated good and with respect. I hope they will get what belong to them. Also remember the love I have for them. I always want the best for my four beautiful childern.

I want my childern to know that I love them and I will do my best to do what it takes to live just for them. If it take me hunders years to do the treatment I will do it to seen their future.

CHAPTER 9

Sometime I wish that I have all the money in the world to give to my childern or buy them what they want. As a single mother it is very hard for me to have ends meet. sometime my older daughter will baker cookies to sell in school to make extra money.

One day I said to my self I went to school to learn how to do hair so why can't I do hair at home to make some extra money. So I went on the internet to make me a business cards. But still it was the same I just straggle in life.

Right now, I want to spend more time with my childern because I don't know when god will call me or when my life will end. I'm just taking it one day at a time to love and care for my beautiful childern. Who knows what tommorrow may bring. No ones life is grantee for tommorrow.

I try to enjoy my life going out and also thinking about geting a breast inplant so that I can feel like a woman again. By me having my breast remove makes me feel less of a woman.

CHAPTER 10

Thank god that I was introduce to two wonderful people at NewYork Presbyterian Hopital. Their names are doctor Kevin Kalinsky and nurse Debbie. Doctor Kalinsky is a doctor who knows his work and treats all his patients with respect. Doctor Kalinsky understands what a person like me is going through. He knows my struggle and pain. Nurse Debbie is also my nurse who takes care of me before my doctor come in to see me. Debbie makes me feel like a normal human being. She is so sweet helpful and god bless Dr. Kalinsky, Nurse Debbie, and their families. God should give them what their heart desire.

All the workers at Doctor Kalinsky's office are very nice and sweet to all their patients who come their to see the doctors and the nurses. Doctor Kalinsky, Nurse Debbie and also everybody in the office are the second people I give thanks to. I want god to be with them where ever they go and give them all a long life to live including their family and friends. these two people was send to me by god almightly they are my angle.

CHAPTER 11

My one and only therapist whom helped me over come my fear also help me to talked about what is bothering me. We talk about how I was dealing with my sickness and what a wonderful mother I was. This threapist helped me in so many ways by listing to me and give me so many advice. I love him and god bless him and his family.

As a cancer patient you have to have faith in your self and the lord. I know that Jehovah will one day heal me from my sickness. Also you should be able to communicate with god by parying and asking him for forgiveness and for him to heal you.

We always want to work so hard to do your treatment so that our childern can blossom into beautiful flowers while growing up. We need to love them more and spend quality time with them.

"Come unto me, all ye that labor and heavy laden, and I will give you rest. Take my yoke upon you, and learn of me For I am meek and lowly in heart, and ye shall find rest unto your souls. For my yoke is easy, and my burden is light."–Matthew 11:28–30

www.ingramcontent.com/pod-product-compliance
Lightning Source LLC
Chambersburg PA
CBHW061224280526
45784CB00006B/2615